Ebola:

The Untold Stories Of Survivors

Gerald Amandu Matua

Gerald Amandu Matua

For more information please contact the author at:

Gerald Amandu Matua
P.O. Box 7782 Kampala, Uganda
Tel: +256 772 522 938 - Uganda
Tel: +968 9982 8042 - Oman
E-mail: gmatua@gmail.com
https://www.facebook.com/amandu.matua

DEDICATION

*This book is dedicated to all survivors of Ebola hemorrhagic fever who have
stood up to the odds of one of humanity's most debilitating diseases!*

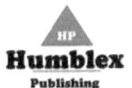

Printed by Create Space, An Amazon.com Company

ISBN-10: 1508981329
ISBN-13: 978-1508981329

Gerald Amandu Matua

CONTENTS

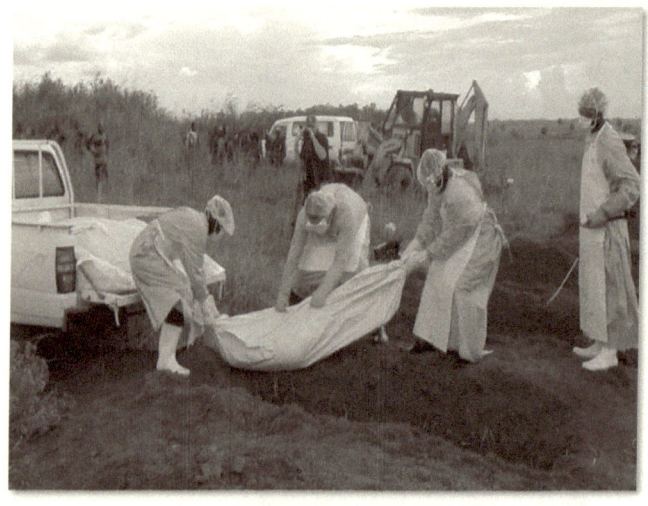

Ferocious Killer: Victims of Ebola being Laid to rest in Gulu, Uganda in 2000

PREFACE

This book is the human story of Ebola, a hemorrhagic disease that ruthlessly affects humans and our "cousins", the great apes – monkey, chimpanzees and the like, inducing acute fever, bleeding tendencies and death within a few days! Ebola outbreaks have continued to occur sporadically since 1976, when the virus was first discovered near River Ebola, in the Democratic Republic of the Congo, then Zaire. Transmitted accidentally to animals or humans by direct contact with the natural reservoir; current research evidence points to species of African fruit bats as playing a major role in aiding transmission process.

In the last 40 years, most of the major Ebola outbreaks have occurred in Africa. Most outbreaks have affected communities in Southern Sudan, the River Congo basin, Uganda and most recently, West Africa. Of all these places, the last twelve years has seen Uganda, one of the East African countries bear the brunt of five outbreaks!

Having witnessed these epidemics and extensively researched the lived experiences of people who came face to face with Ebola within the last 12 years, the author highlights salient features of the human stories that often remain untold. These untold stories date back to 2000 and 2012. These untold stories from Uganda will undoubtedly provide you a unique vantage point from which to better visualize events from the current West African outbreak.

This book is part of the *"Ebola: The Untold Stories"* series that have been carefully designed to bring you deep personal untold stories of surviving Ebola, caring for family members with Ebola as well as being orphaned by Ebola. The unique experiences of men and women widowed by Ebola as well as the silent agonies of health workers - nurses, doctors and others who play critical roles in the fight against Ebola are also included in these series.

Gerald Amandu Matua

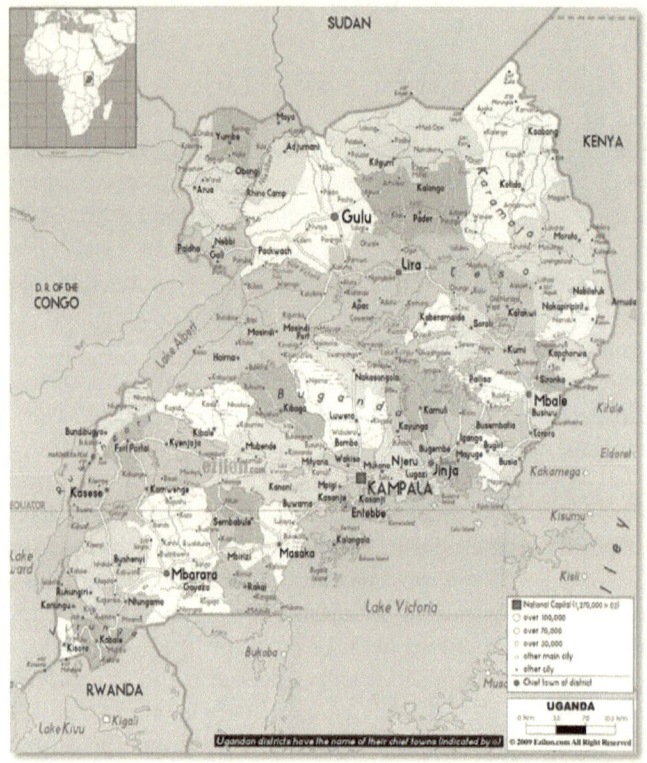

Map of Uganda Showing Main Towns and Countries

Copyright © Ezilon.com, 2009
(Source: http://www.ezilon.com/maps/africa/uganda-maps.html)

1 PROLOGUE
WRESTLING WITH DEATH

Have you ever heard of *"Darkness at Noon"*? Yes! This is how it feels like, when one is told that they have Ebola! The weight is incredible! The news hits them like a ruthless judge's death sentence! And soon crippling fear follows. Victims have described feeling the "earth" below their feet crumbling and their clothes feeling tight upon hearing that inside them is the world's most lethal virus!

Soon sufferers' minds explode with apprehension and hopelessness...unsure what the future holds for them! Then, a few hours later, the physical symptoms of the disease...often pain becomes unbearable, swiftly giving way to despair! The immediate concern becomes, *"Am I going to die or will I survive?"* An Ebola patient's mind suddenly gets filled with endless worries and jeopardy!

Quickly they begin to anticipate death, while hoping to survive this ordeal! For most people, in a matter of days, their normal life freezes still. Uninvited strangers dressed in *"space suits"* secured from head to toe soon appear at their courtyards. Sometimes with armed escort, the sufferers are ordered to board a waiting ambulance...as every spot on which they've stepped is sprayed with Clorox solution!

In the name of limiting further spread of Ebola, victims find themselves being rushed to a place most would rather avoid - the *"isolation ward"* in a designated treatment centre. Unsure if they will ever return home again, they board the ambulance reluctantly…and soon the sirens light up again!

Once the sufferer is admitted to the dreaded isolation unit, their life is ripped apart – their family and friends are forbidden from visiting them for weeks. Owing to the strict infection prevention protocol, the human touch of care seems far removed; at least it feels that way initially.

With time, patients have to get used to caregivers covering their faces securely in protective gear. With all these events occurring rapidly, the Ebola patient feels uprooted from normal life. Suddenly a grisly feeling of loneliness emerges!

As days go by, sufferers begin to experience debilitating physical symptoms – an attack of mercilessly intense headache and body pain grip them from nowhere. It feels like the head is about to split into two halves! The fever persists as muscles and bones ache ruthlessly. The joints decimate, the back hurts and the entire body feels crushed – the feeling is much like being *"run over by a speeding car"*!

In their pain and weakness, patients feel utterly helpless! Their minds are consumed in thoughts… they worry about their families, friends, businesses, jobs and the like! Apprehension loiters relentlessly and is overbearing, especially when patients feel abandoned by health workers.

In the isolation unit, the feeling of hopelessness is re-ignited every time piercing sounds of ambulance sirens burst through to the wards. And this same feeling is re-lived each time a patient dies in the unit! These menacingly loud bellows of ambulance sirens plus the ceaseless deaths constantly remind patients about their own vulnerabilities!

Sometimes, patients are so frightened that they plead with the attending healthcare workers not to leave them alone!

Sometimes it is the attending health workers who are thrown into panic! Such hellish incidences occur when patients become violent, confused or break their quarantine... and begin to move about in the ward. Such freaking sights do not only frighten other patients, but they also put attending health workers' courage to utmost test!

In essence, when patients lose their mind and break loose, so too does hell break loose! Suddenly tension builds in the ward as in a war situation! Nurses and doctors scramble to subdue the wandering patient - some with dripping blood, while others splatter raw feces and vomit across the floor! The scenes can be overwhelming - some caregivers freeze!

For most patients, knowing that even health workers are startled by the illness further deepens their sense of powerlessness. "Even health workers are afraid?", some patients ask as they struggle to come to terms with their new own reality!

Well it is not always bad news! Hope isn't always far – it quickly creeps in whenever caregivers subdue their fear and provide proper care. In most cases treatment consists of administering intravenous fluids, painkillers and antibiotics to treat related symptoms. In the midst of darkness, caregivers' caring actions radiate hope and make patients' realize that they could survive their ordeal with Ebola. In between the lows, patients find strength in spiritual figures and practices – for most prayer offers a formidable support!

With time, some patients are lucky or rather strong enough to overcome the effects of Ebola virus on their vital organs and body systems. As they get better, increasingly they become less fearful about death! Although most patients are still relatively weak, a greater sense of optimism gradually *dilutes* the terror of imminent death as hope rises!

After weeks of waiting, when news of possible survival trickle in, most times survivors are skeptical about the promising laboratory findings. To some such news is *"too good to be true"!* They ask questions like…*"Am I the one going to survive? Is it me who has survived Ebola? Is it true that I am not going to die?* Some breakdown and weep…with tears of joy, while others can't thank God enough for reviving them! Quite often, survivors consider their healing a real miracle!

This point marks an important transition period, with most patients moving away from despair to hope. In the process, some question why they've survived while others - their family and friends didn't! A few others struggle to find meaning in their experience! However, a few more seemingly get *'stuck'*, and continuously whine over the difficulties their association with Ebola has caused them.

This transitory period is uniquely an emotional one and so any psychological support is a major boost! Support from others is critical at this stage, because many patients are still fragile and are yet to fully come to terms with their ordeals. In addition to these uncertainties, many survivors grapple with challenges related to poor appetite, hearing and sight difficulties let alone mental images of suffering!

Grief is also common as survivors lament over the loss of relatives and friends. The fear of death continues to linger on in survivors' minds. Regrettably, recovery process is slow. Moral support is highly recommended at this stage before survivors are discharged from the hospital.

Eventually when survivors are discharged from the isolation units, many find themselves thrown into a *'new'* world - where many feel like *'aliens'* in a world unknown to them! As they return home, usually escorted by surveillance teams, *home coming* is a dream come true for some, while for others, it's marks the beginning of *suffering*. Once home, how survivors are received depends on the level of fear in their community. Often, survivors' relatives are more scared about Ebola than survivors themselves! Many of them notice their relatives and friends are fearful -

some even become suspicious! A potent antiseptic, *Clorox* or *Jik,* as it is locally known suddenly acquires a special status, becoming a *"must have"* companion in every home!

As survivors settle down, whether their homecoming turns out as a joyful or sorrowful event depends on how well their family and community receives them. Where fear is subdued, survivors are received with excitement! The mood is that of celebration. Close friends and relatives gather together in praise of God for sparing their kin's life. At the end of the day, a sumptuous meal crowns the affair.

However, the story is different for others! In homes where fear thrives, survivors get rejected and abandoned, sometimes out rightly! At times, they're disheartened by the cold reception they receive, particularly when they expected they would be warmly received by their relatives. In some cases survivors are openly shunned by relatives!

Where survivors are not welcome, the rejection can be dramatic and far reaching. Some survivors are annihilated from a community they once cherished and called their own! In some instances, village paths get re-drawn as the locals tactfully circumvent the targeted survivors' homes.

In the wider community, the fear of Ebola can be equally crippling. In churches, attendance drops considerably. The usually packed pews remain largely empty. The few who manage to come for worships sit far apart from each other!

Handshakes, during prayer session are quickly abandoned, like any other direct contact with others. The unusual act of nodding to one another becomes *modus operandi* for expressing collegiality during prayer sessions. Priests too are apprehensive and like parishioners, they avoid contact with others. Some priests have used spoons to distribute communion to others, all in the name of avoiding contact.

In mosques, the number of the faithful worshippers reduce drastically too. Unlike in the past, people stand far apart during prayers and avoid making direct contact with one another. In the banks, tellers wear gloves. Like bankers, some market women and shopkeepers also don gloves - all these to ensure that any possible infection is kept at bay!

Public transport also gets deserted. As a safety measure, taxi operators dash off to get gloves and periodically refuse to give lifts to people *'suspected'* to have connection with Ebola, like health workers and hospital workers. These usually "passenger conscious" men suddenly prioritize life over money and become choosy on who boards their cabs!

The free movement of residents from one part of their community to another becomes a contentious matter either officially or through fear motivated actions of vigilantes, who are keen on preventing further spread of the infection.

Such pervasive fear and sometimes government enforced quarantine forces communities to abandon their usual life style, as markets and shops close and businesses grind to a halt!

Such is the state of affairs that lingers on in most Ebola affected areas. The tense atmosphere begins to return to normal, as the epidemic is brought under control. It's only then that survivors' lives gradually normalize!

❧❧

2 CONQUERING DEATH

This is the story of a young Midwife who unknowingly got infected with Ebola in her line of duty. Here is the account of her tribulations and then eventual triumph!

Oh…what a fever it was! I'd no idea whatsoever that the persistent chills that I had were the warning signs of Ebola, a disease that would later, almost claim my life! I hadn't even known that there was already an outbreak and that I'd be among the first to contract Ebola! I imagined that my headache and fever were signs of bout of malaria!

I only realized that I'd Ebola when I was admitted in hospital. Before then, I'd swallowed some analgesics and anti-malarial medications when these symptoms first appeared. I always did so in the past, hoping that I'd soon become better after these meds. I was terribly wrong! This time the nagging pains and the fever wouldn't go away!

Instead, the fever and body ache progressively

worsened. Soon I was weakening by the day! And slowly, I began to worry, especially when the sickness began to interfere with my work. I began to struggle with my work! For days I couldn't find strength to go to work, something unusual of me…I always worked through mild pains! This time I remained home, hoping that I'd soon get better!

Early one morning, after waking up from a *"poor night's sleep"*, I decided that it was time to see a physician later in the day for treatment, because I wasn't improving. Just as I finished bathing in preparation for the visit to the physician, a group of people suddenly arrived and parked outside my home. I could see them clearly through my bedroom window. At this my heart sank! "What is happening here?" I asked myself. Flashes of thoughts dashed through my mind. *"Did somebody do something wrong?"* I contemplated! *"Is there a criminal event?"* I asked myself!

A few seconds later, another vehicle pulled over, this time a hospital ambulance. And four men quickly jumped out - they were dressed up, from head-to-toe in *'space suits'*. I had never seen people dressed like that before! I was petrified when they began to walk towards my house. Furiously, I could hear my heart pounding away! Unexpectedly, I began to choke. There was a lump in my throat and I couldn't breathe! I didn't know what do next!

Then, one of the men called me out by name…"Angela, Angela is that you?" he asked! With my knees trembling almost uncontrollably, "Yes I'm the one", I answered. "Have you been sick lately?" he questioned. And I replied in the affirmative! I even told him that I was actually preparing to go to see a doctor later that morning because of my worsening fatigue, headache and fever!

"Did you take your temperature this morning?" He continued, to which I replied "No I hadn't"… "Take this thermometer and measure your temperature", he instructed, as he handed over to me a thermometer! As instructed, I took my temperature. I told him it was 38.5 degrees Celsius (101.3 degrees Fahrenheit). "You've high fever"… you have to come with us now", he declared!

"Who have you been in touch with lately?" One of them asked! Unsure why these strange looking men were asking me all these unfamiliar questions, I reluctantly replied, "My housemaid and three other colleagues at work and a few other patients whose names I couldn't remember"! Once again and firmly too, the leader ordered, "Pack your clothes and personal effects and come with us right away"!

As I packed my belongings, some of the men started spraying around my house. "Where is your bedroom and bathroom?" They asked me! "We need to spray there too" another added! "Go ahead and spray wherever you want to", I retorted angrily! I was clearly upset. I couldn't understand why a team of strange men were doing weird things in my home, early in the morning with no clear explanations! What annoyed me most was how guarded they were with their explanations. They spoke little. "They must be up to something wicked", I thought as I packed!

By then completed overpowered and feeling depressed, with barely any energy to spare, I couldn't resist anymore! I decided that I'd cooperate with the strangers nonetheless. Bizarrely, whereas I was quite upset with these men, I was equally relieved that they'd offered to take me to the hospital. "Maybe it was my luck", I ruminated silently.

As we left home, the sirens of the ambulance violently pierced through the quietness of the morning. It must have been about 8:00 o'clock. The sky was clear and the tropical sun shone brightly as the morning breeze shook the leaves of plants along the way!

My neighbors were bewildered as the ambulance dashed away hurriedly. The expressions of wonder were clearly written on each of their faces! Like me, they had no clue what was going on with me…much less that there was an Ebola outbreak!

What was clear to all the neighbors was that a team from the district hospital came in suddenly and *"whisked"* away a Midwife well known to them, and that was me! They much like me didn't understand why, as was clearly written on their fear riddled faces! They appeared no less than shocked! Soon, I lost sight of my neighborhood as we sped fast through the village roads, raising clouds of dust!

When we arrived at the hospital, the men escorted me straight to a strange section of the hospital unknown to me, made up of tarpaulin (grey canvas) and surrounded by a short orange plastic fence, slightly over a meter high!

"Why do you bring me to this place?" I asked.
"This is the isolation ward", their leader replied!
"Why isolation ward?" I inquired.
"There is an outbreak of a strange disease", he said!

As I entered this strange place, which I eventually realized was an isolation ward, I noticed that there was already one other patient in the isolation room. He was a middle aged man, about 50 years of age! Everything looked strange as I gazed around and out through the plastic window of the tarpaulin. In a distance, the hospital was quiet and looked abandoned! You could hardly see people move around in the compound as they did in the past!

The isolation ward was far removed from other hospital wards. I felt isolated from the rest of the world. Suddenly, a feeling of uncertainty ran over me. Unsure of what to expect and what would happen to me next, I sat quietly on one of the beds nearby and just waited!

It was an old bed, placed right next to the plastic window, dressed with an aging grey-white blanket and white supple medium-sized pillow! A small metallic bedside locker was the only other thing I had, except for the IV stand that stood next to the bed. As I sat down, I pondered wearily what the future held for me - would I die or would I survive, I wondered quietly as I waited to see what'd happen next!

Minutes later, a group of people entered the ward. "Now these must be doctors and nurses" I said to myself! I was right! They too were dressed in white '*space suits*'. They walked straight towards me. "We have come to take your blood for laboratory test", said one of them. And then another one told me gently, "There is a serious disease outbreak around, and we don't yet know what it is", he explained. "And we request that you to corporate with us" he added. I was silent. "It must really be a serious disease", I thought to myself!

As I contemplated about this outbreak, one of them, talking in a familiar voice, began to explain: "A few days ago a clinician working in this hospital died of a strange disease and we're trying to investigate it"! Suddenly my senses woke up! I quickly realized that I'd actually attended the funeral of this very clinician! I became more alert. I'd even cared for her in the antenatal clinic where I worked as Midwife, looking after her and other mothers unaware that she or even others could have been infected!

At once, I thought it must be a serious disease then...perhaps even an infectious disease outbreak! As they explained her symptoms, I could see striking similarity. Then it began to sink in my mind, albeit slowly why these fellows were dressed in such attire and were acting rather eccentrically!

As my mind went round and round in bewilderment, I was requested to provide a sample of my blood for lab tests! I obliged and some sample was soon taken off. And then they told me that I'd be observed for a few more days as they waited for the results of my blood tests.
And off they went!

Time stood still! I spent the rest of the day as I deliberated with great difficulty what this strange outbreak might turn out to be! As the sun set and the evening breeze fought its way into the plastic isolation ward...I began to feel cold! Unlike the receding rays, my fever and headache only got worse! A little while later, calm returned and the raging fever like the throbbing headache subsided! And off I slept…and day one was all but gone!

The next day, I began to feel weaker and weaker. I had sharp abdominal pains that would come and then go away. It quickly became an uncomfortable rhythm. I was five months pregnant by then! The painful rhythm soon became a contraction. I became increasingly worried. I was gripped by fear…"I hope something terrible doesn't happen to my pregnancy!" I trembled as I prayed fervently.

Surely, as I'd feared, after about an hour or so, I began to bleed. "I am bleeding", I cried out loudly! The pain was unbearable! It was the worst pain I have experienced in my entire life! The bleeding was terrifying…even for a midwife like me! I cried and shouted for help, but to my surprise no one came to my rescue! It was as if the health workers never heard any of my cries!

For hours, I cried for help! And in agony, I had puddles of sweat running through my body. I was drenched in sweat. I was all by myself with no one to help me. I was completely exhausted.
The unending contraction,
and the crying took the better part of my energy.
I was distressed!

And soon, the worst happened!
Suddenly, I felt the contractions intensifying violently!
Lo and behold! The fetus rushed out!
Unbelievably, I'd lost my precious baby!
The contractions were no more, except for the bleeding!

After a while, when I looked at the gestational sac, I noticed it was incomplete. At once, I knew that the placenta had remained inside me and this was pretty dangerous! I knew I'll probably bleed to death if nothing is done. Momentarily, I was paralyzed and overran by fear!

I felt cold shivers running down my spine as I searched for solutions. My mind was in a terrible time race! At once, and almost in a flash, I told myself, "I'll try to deliver the placenta"! Frantically, I started pulling out the remaining piece of the sac...but then, unluckily it broke! Without even realizing it, I let out a loud cry! "Can somebody help me', 'please someone help me'..." I cried!

I continued to wail loudly! But there was no response from the health workers.

I was desperate.

The bleeding continued...

After a while, I heard a group of doctors and nurses entering the ward. By this time I was feeling drowsy and exceedingly feeble. With all my strength, I shouted: "I've lost my baby and I'm bleeding badly, can somebody help me?" I'd imagined that my howling would turn things around for me. I was wrong...rather the reverse happened!

To the contrary, my loud cries scared away the team – both doctors and nurses! When some of them drew closer to see what I was talking about, they saw I was soaked in blood. They were very astounded and pulverized by the sight! I've never seen nurses or doctors that petrified!

With a trembling voice, one of them yelled, "She might have Ebola"! They all froze. None of them dared to come any closer to help me. And they all retreated and left the ward in great hurry, without even touching me!

And the bleeding continued...

I became weaker and weaker.

I couldn't even lift my head off the bed.

And...bit by bit, I felt my "*spirit*" depart.

I could remember no more!

Surely....and slowly, I drifted into coma...

The following day, when I became conscious again, I noticed that I was still covered in a pool of blood. Luckily, the bleeding had stopped. And when I checked myself, I noticed the placenta was still inside me. I didn't know what to do! And so I called out again...

After a while, two people, I guess nurses soon came to me and then handed over to me some pills and told me to swallow them! Soon after swallowing the pills, I promptly told them that I was still bleeding! But they refused to pay attention to what I was telling them. What surprised me most was the fact that they both acted like I hadn't told them anything! Both of them simply ignored my plea for help. And none of them dared to touch me! And shortly after, they left the ward!

I was left desperate...

"I'll die here if I don't do anything", I told myself! After a while, I gathered some strength and decided it was time to call my husband...yes, I thought firmly! But there was a problem! My hands were covered in blood and so I couldn't dial his number. I had to find a way... I decided to instruct a fellow patient to call my husband on phone and ask him to rush to the hospital immediately to come to my rescue! I wanted him to plead with the hospital authorities so that they would assist me. I'd tried several times to get help, but all my pleas were without success!

And yet I could see death right before my eyes. Still bleeding, I deteriorated and went into coma again...

And when I woke up the next day, I noticed that I was lying down on the floor. I'd fallen off the bed and had spent the entire night on the floor. Although the bleeding had stopped, I still felt pretty weak. I couldn't find enough energy to get back to bed! And so I sat down on the floor next to my bed and rested for a while!

Moments later, a group of doctors and nurses entered the ward and saw me seated on the floor. I hadn't gathered enough strength to lift myself back to bed. This time it seems luck was on my side. All dressed in white *"space suits"* one of them called me by name, "Angela", "Angela"...he said, "Don't be afraid", he continued. "We have come to help you!" he declared as they drew close!

I was surprised to see how relaxed they all looked this time, it seems, the apprehension had melted away! They all looked very confident and no more frightened. Holding each of my hands, two of them, both men helped me up and then back onto my bed. Unexpectedly, I felt accepted! After cleaning me up, the team leader confidently announced that they were now going to remove the placenta. When I heard this, a cloud of hope swiftly enveloped me. "I will survive this disease", I declared! And a spurt of energy quickly rushed through me. I felt relieved!

Finally, the retained placenta was removed... I was then asked to insert a tablet to stop the bleeding. And...like they told me, the bleeding stopped soon after!

Everything seemed to take a new turn. After the team removed the placenta, their leader told me that they had my lab results. And in a surprisingly calm manner, while holding my hand, he told me I'd tested positive for Ebola!

I wasn't shocked either. Confident that I was already recovering, I wasn't worried that much! But what really surprised me was the response of the medical team. I'd expected a fear-dominated reaction, but to my surprise, their reaction was very calm. They were mostly at ease with me. They even assured me that "*my blood was strong*". "You have good chances of making it", they assured me! "We'll give you all the necessary treatment and you'll be ok", another one of them declared!

After the team left the ward, I was asked to continue with treatment, which involved no more than pain killers, antibiotics and intravenous fluids. This moment on, my worries reduced drastically. This time round, much more relaxed than previously, I continued with my treatment regimen and I prayed and hoped for the best outcome!

Slowly I began to recover. Day by day I felt better. Even though I was still weak, I wasn't horrified anymore! Then I didn't fear death.
I became firm.
"I won't die", I'd tell myself.
I didn't know why, but I was confident about recovering from Ebola!

Several days later, a team of doctors came to see me as part of the routine medical checkups. However, this time I noticed that they acted with some bit of excitement.

"What are these fellows up to?" I pondered silently!

As the team approached me, I could see the team leader was clearly excited. *"Angela, Angela...*we have good news for you", he declared in a husky voice! To this day, I remember this moment very clearly. "In a few days, we shall discharge you", he added. "After just a few more tests you'll surely be on your way home", he declared with unusual confidence! Instantly, I felt hope surrounding me!

With all these affirmations, I began to ask myself, "Am I the one going to survive?" "Is it true that I've survived Ebola?" "This must be a miracle" I declared! I couldn't believe at first. It was simply too much for me. I continued to thank God for healing me. "Dear God, please make me survive this illness, I don't want to die", I kept on fervently imploring God!

For days, I waited for final laboratory results before I was discharged home from the isolation ward. Doctors, nurses and counsellors continued to encourage me as I waited for these results. They'd tell me "you need to eat and drink a lot". And with their support and constant assurance my optimism grew as I waited for the results!

A couple of day later, the results came. It was all clear! I was now Ebola free! I was then congratulated by the medical staff in the isolation unit and permitted to go home, accompanied by the surveillance team members.

Finally, after several weeks under quarantine and tight restrictions I was finally on my way home. I started feeling nostalgic as the ambulance left the hospital gate...my journey back home had begun. I felt strong and confident and looked forward to the new life ahead of me!

When I arrived home, I was surprised to find how hysterical and fearful people had become! My neighbors were drowning in fear. I could see they were overtly nervous. Out of fear, many people abandoned age old expressions of friendships and collegiality like handshakes and physical embraces. There were people walking around wearing gloves! Even our local market and shops closed.

Fear and anxiety were palpable and everywhere you looked! The locals couldn't mix freely with one another; and all forms of social cohesion came to an abrupt end!

Luckily for me, when the news of my return spread, the locals didn't run away from me! I felt accepted.

Many relatives and friends were happy to see me return alive. "You survived because of your good deeds", some remarked. "God healed you because of the good things you did to us", others reiterated.

The caring attitude shown by my relatives and friends was gratifying! In retrospect, this experience has made me to realize the importance of helping others – it has even made me to love my job more!

3 THE EBOLA FUGITIVE

*This is the true story of a middle aged businessman
who escaped from an Ebola unit and caused serious
pandemonium as epidemic control scouts frantically
combed surrounding villages until he was captured and
safely returned to his "new home" - the isolation unit!*

In late November 2000, as I went about my usual work of
shop keeping, I began to feel feverish! Within hours the
fever intensified. "What might be happening to me?" I
wondered. I even told my wife that I wasn't feeling alright.

Soon I developed a strange headache that wouldn't
go away; followed by striking coldness, which I'd never
experienced before! "I must have malaria", I thought. But
when I went to a nearby clinic, the test was negative.

My pains continued throughout that day and by dusk the feeling of coldness was overwhelming! "I'll fight back", I declared! And so I dressed up heavily to beat the cold chill. I wore a very heavy jacket, on top of two warm shirts and a coat. By night the coldness intensified. It was so bad that I was forced to cover myself with four blankets in all.

Despite dressing up in unusually thick clothing, I still felt extremely cold. I felt as if I was sleeping outside the house in cold weather! "Why I am feeling this cold?" I kept wondering! "What kind of disease is this?" I thought to myself! "Could this be a kind of malaria that doesn't respond to treatments?" I wondered.

The next day, just as the cold seemed to subside, the fever intensified and my muscles began to ache mercilessly! A little while later, I began to feel body weakness which got me worrying!

And so I began to retrace my set steps...

Then, I remembered that I was feeling much like my land lord's daughter whom I'd taken to hospital the previous week. I also recalled that while I was tending to the sick girl, I'd visited a friend in the same hospital who'd been admitted with high fever and persistent body aches.

"May be I've a similar disease", I contemplated quietly in my mind! Then, I quickly recalled how one of the two, the businesswoman lay helpless in her hospital bed. I remember asking her, "What are you doing here?"

She was very sick and her lips were cracked and her eyes sunk deep into the skulls! She struggled to breathe let alone talk! I remember, she had beads of sweat rolling down her forehead and the look of helplessness was written everywhere on her face!

"I must have contracted an illness from these two ladies!" I concluded. I then remembered that I'd been in contact with both of them. At this point, I recalled how I'd carried the landlord's daughter to the hospital and later how I leaned against the businesswoman's hospital bed while I talked to her. As I tried to understand the genesis of my stubborn muscle pains, high fevers and splitting headache, especially how I could've contracted the illness, my past interaction with the two patients continuously replayed in my mind! My mind was racing wildly!

As I recalled my interactions with the two patients: the businesswoman and the landlords' daughter, I noticed with stark similarity that my symptoms matched theirs, especially that of the business lady.

I recall she had pounding headache and sore throat which was exceedingly painful. In fact her headache was so severe that she'd hold her frontal bone as she spoke to me!

Like her, I was struggling with very similar set of symptoms of pain and body weakness and the like!

With time, the headache and the weakness increased. I felt terrible pain all over my body. I began to vomit and pass out bloody diarrhea, which unfortunately wouldn't stop, despite treatment!

I was terrified, sore and heartbroken! Later that evening, I collapsed. Scared to their bones, my family rushed me to the district hospital immediately!

When I arrived in the hospital, they revived me and started me on some intravenous fluids. I felt better but the coldness still persisted. I'd feel very cold and yet my temperature was always around 38 to 40 degrees Celsius (100 to 104 degrees Fahrenheit). I'd sweated copiously and my throat dried out. Swallowing became problematic. I couldn't eat well. And so I lost a lot of weight!

Almost after a week in hospital, doctors hadn't identified my sickness! They didn't know precisely what I was suffering from or what my problem was despite taking several blood samples for lab analysis.

What was certain is that my symptoms continued to increase! A while later, I developed hiccups which lasted for 3 days, followed by dry cough and sharp chest pains!

Unsure of what I was suffering from the doctors continue to give me fluids and some pain medications.

Then one day, the unthinkable happened! It was about 10:00 am when I saw a group of people covered from head to toe, heading straight to my ward. When I examined their movements closely, they looked terrified. "Why are these people here and why are they acting like these?" I asked!

When the group entered the ward, they called out for our attention. Then, hell broke loose! Shortly their leader announced that the disease that I and several others in the ward had been suffering from was in fact, *Ebola* hemorrhagic fever.

At once, I knew my life had cracked open, because Ebola had killed hundreds of people in Zaire and the Sudan, our immediate neighboring countries to the west and the north.

Although we were assured that all care would be taken to look after us, anxiety still built up steadily - some health workers who'd by then been looking after us for a couple of weeks simply froze!

Fear was evident and everyone looked scared - doctors, nurses and patients all alike. Momentarily, the entire ward went silent! It was as if nobody was there!

The news of an Ebola outbreak quickly spread throughout the entire hospital. In a little while, I saw patients and their relatives running away…some patients fleeing with IV fluid bottles hanging loose from their arms!

I'd never seen people that hysterical! Many patients fled like they'd never been sick before…simply because they couldn't stand sharing the same hospital with Ebola patients. And for this level of terror, most patients seemed to get better all at once!

Unfortunately, I was one of those patients who couldn't run away, because I'd already tested positive for the deadly Ebola virus.

This revelation devastated me totally. I was in great shock and feared the worst. I worried I'd never see my family again! I thought I wouldn't make it!

Although I was terribly scared from the inside, I tried to present a strong face. I told myself "I will overcome this disease"! I couldn't help, but think about my wife and children. Soon the fear overwhelmed my defenses!

Seeing how scared I was, the nurses and doctors encouraged me to adopt a positive mindset. Despite their support, I couldn't help but think about death, because patients were dying one after another, before my eyes!

These almost unstoppable deaths frightened me to the point of insanity! It was unbearable!

And before long, I lost my mind and I didn't know what was happening to me and where I was! I'd gone nuts!

I was later told that I had become very aggressive to everyone, and in rage, I even tore off my IV lines. After this episode, I escaped from the ward and wandered off causing pandemonium wherever I went!

The surveillance team reportedly gave a chase and dragged me back to the isolation ward! It was after then that I regained my mind!

After recovering from the episode of mental confusion, I felt very thirsty. My body was constantly hot and I sweated copiously. There was a time when I couldn't even urinate for two straight days...my body was dry!

It's then that I decided to drink lots! I could take up to five liters of oral rehydration solution daily. I continued to drink lots despite being on intravenous fluids therapy!

I drank lots of fluids because I knew these were my only treatments...sort of what would keep me alive! I knew I'd to drink to stay alive because my diarrhea wouldn't stop... I even thought I'd lose the battle to Ebola, because on a number of days, I had many motions!

There was one particular moment when I thought I'd not survive to see the next day. That day, I'd passed lots of bloody diarrhea and was extremely weak. I was worried about my condition. I wasn't even sure I'd remain alive, more so, after witnessing two patients adjacent to me deteriorating rapidly and dying right before my very eyes!

Before they died, both patients started bleeding profusely through their nose and mouth. I became even more terrified when one of them, an elderly man chocked as he vomited blood and later died, while the other patient a teenager slipped and fell off his bed as he breathed his last.

That was one of the most terrifying things I'd seen in my entire life! I was frightened to my bones!

From that moment onwards, I knew when people started bleeding or vomiting blood like the two had, it meant that their time would soon be over!

Sadly, the terrifying story didn't just end there! I was frightened once more when the burial team came to put the corpses into body bags. Witnessing the burial team spraying the corpses with Clorox solution and then zipping them up very tightly in body bags scared me enormously!

After seeing all this, I feared that I might be the next. Immensely petrified, I implored God to spare my life. I couldn't sleep. It is a night I'll never forget! I thought I'd die before the morning light. It was my longest night ever!

While I survived that gritty night, I wasn't sure I'd escape death as many had by now perished... and some I witnessed personally. For days, I was apprehensive. I feared I might deteriorate and then die like others had!

As days passed, I gradually became stronger although some fear still persisted. I guess the fluids and pain killers had started helping me! I felt progressively better. I was told to keep drinking and eating aggressively to regain my lost weight. Additional samples of blood were taken from me for lab analysis and I was told to wait for the outcome.

After almost two weeks of waiting, the final results came. And providentially, my fears of death ended because I'd tested negative for Ebola virus.

Suddenly, weeks of waiting had ended...I was declared Ebola free; given a certificate indicating I'd healed and I was permitted to return home!

This was a special moment that I have come to appreciate. At that moment, I felt a very heavy yoke that

I'd been carrying for weeks was suddenly removed from my neck. This burden just vanished and instantly I felt well again! I felt a new dawn had opened in my life!

Overcoming death from Ebola is the best thing that ever happened to me. I was thankful to everyone who cared for me. After weeks of isolation in the wards I couldn't wait to catch up with lost time with my family.

For all these weeks my family couldn't visit me and so I badly longed to see them!

When the surveillance team escorted me home; I found my wife and children anxiously waiting to receive me. I could see they were overjoyed to see me again. I fought back my tears as my wife and children embraced me. They all wept openly as we cuddled each other. This moment meant a lot to me and it still does today! What an awesome reunion…

As the heat of the moment cooled down…so did my happiness. I quickly realized that my happiness was short lived!

While my homecoming was a source of joy for my family, the neighbors' reaction was the opposite. My return renewed a spirit of fear in the neighborhood. Momentarily, neighbors began to avoid me and my family.

At some point, they threatened my children and wife with violence if they insisted on fetching water from the shared village borehole. Some local shops denied us their goods for fear of infection.

Wherever we went, they called us by the name "*Ebola*" and this would send people in frenzy. Neighbors couldn't mix with us like it was before Ebola!

A fortnight after discharge from hospital, I thought it was time to resume work in the shop. I didn't know that I'd soon be in for a rude shock!

Soon I realized that I could hardly make any sales because people were afraid of me. The situation was so bad. Whenever unsuspecting people bought items from my shop they would sometimes return these items and demand for a refund of their money. And their reason was always, "I don't want to get your Ebola!"

I'd be devastated whenever I heard such comments! It made me feel like I'd willfully "hidden" Ebola in the goods I was selling.

This is how I was humiliated now and then, both by people I knew and those I didn't!

It soon became clear to me that my pains hadn't just ended yet…soon it dawned on me that the weeks of suffering I'd endured in the isolation ward weren't as painful as those that waited for me outside!

In the community, the reaction to the epidemic was equally hysterical. The people were consumed by fear and anxiety…and it spread!

At a funeral, mourners undressed themselves and abandoned their clothes at the graveside and fled stark naked after realizing that the deceased had probably died of Ebola! It was their way of keeping safe!

The fear of infection in the community was unimaginable. The mere mention of the word *'Ebola'* wreaked *havoc.* Not only were the local citizens petrified; too were the notorious Lord's Resistance Army rebels who'd earned themselves a reputation for abducting civilians.

News of the outbreak prompted them to display unusual cowardice when they released over 40 recent abductees. It was clear that the fear of infection moved these hard-hearted rebels as much as it did the civilians!

Contracting Ebola has affected me in many ways. I still feel a lot of pain in my chest and I've frequent unexplained headaches.

My sight and hearing have been affected too. I cannot even read for long these days similar to being unable to carry heavy objects as I always did before Ebola.

With my wife, things are not okay! I sometimes exchange unpleasant words with my wife! "Why"? The reason is simple: I'm no longer what I used to be in bed;

the erection is there, but I find I cannot perform to the wife's satisfaction! Besides, I don't have much physical strength. I also forget a lot these days; I've difficulty remembering where I place objects. And this affects me and my business!

Financially, Ebola has made me poor. I lost many of my personal belongings during the outbreak. There was a policy to destroy by burning or burying all things we had touched...including beddings, clothes and other personal effects that were believed to provide a safe haven for Ebola!

In the early days of the outbreak, the Ebola scouts went to suspected patients' homes and destroyed all what they thought was the "breeding ground of Ebola". This left me desperately poor.

I had to start life over again! Some teams were so vigilant in clearing the victims' homes...and this made us to lose many valuables. Awkwardly, the external support to help us replace these items has been very slow!

Nowadays reflecting on the experience, I can say that Ebola has created a scar in my mind that is difficult to heal! I am still struggling to get over the painful experience.

These days, whenever I fall sick, I still find myself automatically recalling and re-living the agonies in the hospital and at home at the time.

Frankly speaking, Ebola striped me of "my old self". I've continued to suffer the after effects of the Ebola attack for several months after surviving the illness!

4 WAITING TO DIE EVERY DAY

This is the story of a midwife who contracted Ebola when duty called – she'd struggled to save the life of a pregnant woman who bled profusely and was at the verge of death!

When I got infected, I didn't know that the relentless headache, fever, vomiting and diarrhea were related to Ebola. I knew that I could have possibly contracted Ebola after I was transferred to a referral hospital in the city far away. This was after nearly two weeks of illness and after failing to respond to all manner of orthodox treatments!

Earlier on when the fever and the body aches began, my reaction was…perhaps I've got some complicated malaria! But then, I wouldn't improve despite medication.

Instead, I became weaker and weaker. A few days later, I became so weak that and I was unable to move out of bed. For days, I couldn't even report to work.

When I failed to report to work, my colleagues got so concerned because this was unusual. And so that evening they came home to check on me.

When they arrived, I struggled to get up to entertain them.

Seeing how frail I was, my colleagues immediately called for an ambulance which rushed me to the nearest hospital for urgent medical attention.

And when we arrived at the hospital, I was admitted right away and put on IV fluids. By then, I was running a high fever and started vomiting soon after we arrived. I felt exhausted!

The doctors thought that I had complicated malaria or something of the sort. Some thought of cholera because of the loose stools. I was given quinine to treat the suspected malaria and antibiotics to counter the cholera!

I continued to deteriorate rapidly throughout the night. And the vomiting too worsened! This time it was blood stained. With these unusual symptoms, I began to ask myself questions like, "Why I am not responding to any treatment?" Even the doctors and nurses treating me looked worried. They were clearly confused, much like me!

A day earlier, I'd I arrived while talking normally…and now, a few hours later I was too weak to even talk!

"We are referring you", the physician-in-charge quickly confirmed!

Shortly, I was on a 4 hour's journey by road to a specialist hospital in the city for better treatment. The ambulance driver tried his best to make the ride as smooth as he could!

Hours later, we arrived at the referral hospital. I still had high fever but the vomiting had stopped. Shortly after, I was given some IV fluids and antibiotics. Also, samples of blood and stool were taken for laboratory investigations.

My first night in the new hospital was largely uneventful.

The following day, the lab results once again showed no evidence of malaria or cholera. Unsure of what I was suffering from the attending physician prescribed for me a second line of anti-malarial treatment with antibiotics.

On the third day, as I lay down on my back, with my mind wandering about aimlessly, I heard the normal TV programming being interrupted. *"Breaking News"*, announced the anchor! When I heard this, I slowly turned towards the TV set to get a glimpse of the breaking news!

"An Ebola outbreak has been confirmed in Kibale district in Western Uganda", the anchor announced!

"Health authorities have indicated that most patients are presenting with symptoms of headache, fever and occasional diarrhea", she continued.

In a second, I thought, "Kibale is where I come from and I seem to have all these symptoms, could it be that I have Ebola?

Immediately, my mind went into a wild roller coaster ride! "Where could I have got this disease"? I asked myself as I scanned through my patients!

Then unexpectedly I remembered that, a young woman had been brought it, bleeding profusely with an incomplete abortion.

I also recalled that an attendant had told me that several other people in their village had died under unclear circumstances and a few others were still sick! When I had inquired about the cause of the deaths, she'd told me the villagers thought someone was bewitching the family!

That was where the story had ended and then I continued with my work.

Uh! When I remembered these words, I could now make the connections. "The miscarriage and the bleeding from her nose and mouth must have been due to Ebola" I reasoned!

I could now see how I probably contracted the illness. I remembered treating the pregnant woman like any other mother - without any special protective items apart from simple gloves. I didn't even use a face mask! The miscarriage and the unusual bleeding from her nose and mouth somehow didn't catch my attention!

With an Ebola outbreak confirmed, I knew straight away that I could have been exposed to the virus. I now expected the worse! I knew Ebola couldn't be treated and so I waited to die!

And true to my fears, a call soon came through from Kibale where I worked! "Where are you?" The caller inquired. "We need to take blood samples from you", he insisted. And after a while, a group of doctors dressed in white overalls from head-to-toe came up to me!

I knew straight away something wasn't right. And one of them told me directly, "We have come to take your blood for lab analysis because of an Ebola outbreak in Kibale, where you came from!"

We want to be sure that you weren't exposed to Ebola", he added, as he carefully drew the blood sample from my left arm. I could see they were scared!

Three days later, two of the people who'd taken my blood returned with a few other people. They were all covered, from head-to-toe, in 'Ebola attire'.

I felt something was wrong... and I was right! Their message was, "all the laboratory tests show that you've been exposed to Ebola"!

This announcement hit me like a bombshell. I was utterly devastated and confused! I was so upset.
While I suspected that I may've been exposed to Ebola when caring for patients, I was shocked by the confirmation of the illness.

Like me, this announcement frightened everyone – my sisters, the nurses and the doctors who'd been looking after me!

Everybody was speechless and visibly unsettled!
Out of fear, a doctor even tried to persuade her colleagues to discharge me prematurely!

I remember she suggested, "I think we should return her to Kibale, since we are not going to manage her here!" She said in a trembling voice!

Momentarily, I saw all the nurses and doctors leaving my room - one after another and in total silence! They were clearly downtrodden! Just outside my room I heard them lamenting.

One of them exclaimed repeatedly "We're finished!" We're finished!" Like them, my mind was flooded with all sorts of thoughts. I was bewildered!

Uncertain about the future, my mind wandered endlessly - my thoughts oscillated between despair and hope; and between death and survival!

I feared the worst could happen! But most of all, I felt sorry for those who'd cared for me, especially the nurses and doctors and my siblings.

Like the health workers, my siblings too feared that they'd been contaminated.

Shortly after the announcement and as the doctors left the room, my elder sister asked me, "Sister, now since you've Ebola and you know that Ebola spreads, what we are going to do?" I think she really wanted to say: "Now that I'd Ebola, would it not be wise to let her leave?"

Not surprisingly, while my elder sister was in serious "emotional dire straits".

But, to the contrary, my younger sister surprised me when she declared, "I will never be afraid of you sister... no matter what, I'll take care of you!"

Regardless of what they said, I felt sorry for both of my sisters. And fearing that I may have already infected my siblings, I decided that they wouldn't touch me anymore!

"I'd rather die alone", I told myself! As a precaution, I stopped both of them from touching me. I'd refuse them to bathe me!

And so I waited to die...

I waited to die because I was convinced that my death was imminent. I resorted to lie only in one position in the bed until my final moments arrived...!

Frozen and anticipating imminent death, I prayed to God to show mercy and spare my sisters... and only take

me, if that would save them! I'd surrendered my life…
And I patiently waited to die!

With time, each day I woke up alive, I'd ask God to
keep me alive for the rest of that day. I wanted to survive,
but I doubted if I'd be able to fight on! "Will I really
survive"? I'd ask! Sometimes I'd comfort myself by
reasoning that, "the antibiotics and the IV fluids I'd taken
might heal me".

And so, my confidence began to surge! "I think I'll
survive since I've already spent many days without dying",
I'd say to calm my wildly racing mind, each day I remained
alive!

Day by day, hour by hour, I began to feel better.

Gradually I became hopeful that I would survive! I
started feeling good, especially after several assurances
from counselors, doctors and nurses.

They would tell me, "You are not going to die". Some
would say: "Your days are running fast and you'll soon be
declared Ebola free, so just keep on taking your meds!"
For wanting to survive, I did oblige!

True to their pledge, I started feeling better, both
mentally and physically. I started gaining energy and
became more hopeful, day after day.

I'd say, "If I was to die, I would've already died by
now". "Since I seem to be gaining energy, I think I'll not
die", I'd soothe my fears! And steadily my confidence
grew. I thought that I was now on the way to recovery!

Soon I started sending for newspapers! I became
curious. I desperately wanted to know what was being
published about Ebola and how life was outside my
hospital room, where I had been confined for weeks.

Once, I read a special issue article that said, "…if an
Ebola patient is managed in time by treating their fever,
diarrhea and vomiting, they had good chance of survival".

This discovery made my confidence soar by leaps and
bounds. With this knowledge I told myself, "I think I will
survive"!

Ironically you'd say, aware that I could be on my way to survival, I became overly emotional. I started crying; may be these were cries of joy! I felt exceedingly good.

I asked myself repeatedly "Who am I to survive Ebola?", "How can I survive despite the blood I touched?" "How come I've survived and yet many others have died?" I pondered!

With no answers to the question of why I survived while many others didn't, with great fervor I began to praise God. "I could only have survived because God wanted me to do more work", I'd rationalize!

I remember even pledging, "God if you make me to survive Ebola, I'll go and fulfill your work. I'll return to serve your people in Kibale!" I'd pray to God whenever it was possible, almost unceasingly!

I didn't know why I did so. As I got better, I'd see myself as if I had God's favor… as if I was next to God! It was a strange feeling!

I was elated and incessantly thanked God for healing me! I was also grateful to the doctors and nurses for their care that made me to recover from Ebola!

With time I got better and better and I was eventually discharged! When I returned home, I got mixed reception. Some people feared me, while others received me gladly.

The cowardly would ask me, "Are you really okay before we greet you?" I am sure, what they were really asking me was, "Are you sure you won't infect us with your Ebola?"

Some relatives were pretty gross, others requested that I should go back to the hospital and only return to them when I was sure I was completely healed!

I would always insist that I was completely healed. And whenever I realized they didn't believe me, I'd promptly show them the certificate that declared me "Ebola free"!

Its only when they saw the hospital stamps and signatures, that they'd greet me happily. Others would turn around; smile sheepishly and then apologize for having been very critical!

With time most family members became comfortable with me, except a few others who kept their distance. They continued being cautious. They'd ask me questions like, "Are you truly healed or you could still have Ebola?" Such people upset me so much!

The one thing that strengthened me throughout this period was the unconditional love and acceptance my husband showed me! His acceptance strengthened me a lot and made me to withstand all the disappointments and rejections from the uncaring relatives!

I felt reassured when I knew that my husband wasn't scared of me! "I am ready to die with you" he insisted. "I can't forsake you because you've Ebola", he declared! "If we are to die, then we shall die together", he'd insist!

My husband's reaction was way beyond what I'd expected of him...and this made me feel good. But his sisters-in-laws weren't that comfortable with me, they were apprehensive!

After several weeks of recovery at my village, I returned to my place of work in Kibale.

When I arrived, surprisingly, the locals received me well. My colleagues were happy to see me because rumor had it that I had died.

When they saw me alive many mobbed me excitedly! Instead, it was me who hesitated to touch them because I wasn't accustomed to handshakes anymore, following months of isolation.

I had become accustomed to avoiding getting into contact with people. I had to work actively towards overcoming this impediment!

As I resumed work, I'd to complete some administrative procedures which required my personal file.

But there was a problem! My official file was missing. And it wasn't where it was supposed to be. And so the search for my file began! "Where could my file be?"

I wondered! We continued with the frantic search.

Eventually we discovered that my file was tucked away among that of deceased staff members!

I was shocked by this discovery. "How can these fellows classify my file among the dead?" I asked? It then occurred to me that the rumors of my death had spread widely.

With a sigh of relief, I picked up my file. I couldn't help but I kept wondering silently; "Here I am, with my file placed amongst the dead and yet I am alive!

"What a miracle this must be!" I was grateful to God for being alive!

And when I pondered more deeply about this discovery, I realized that being declared dead, while in fact still alive quickened my resolve to recover and get back onto my feet!

As my journey to recovery continued, the encouragement and support I received from my friends and family, including phone calls and visits made me to feel loved and strong. Above all it empowered me to return to normal life.

I cherished every aspect of such support because Ebola didn't leave me the same; it destroyed a big part of me! To this day I still cry whenever I recall my ordeals with Ebola!

In part I still cherish support from others is because of the several after effects of Ebola that have persisted to this day despite having been declared Ebola free several months earlier.

I still have weaknesses in my thinking, let alone my general health. I'm not all that healed yet. I'm very forgetful these days; I particularly forget about physical objects such as phones and bags. On many occasions, this weakness has made me to lose bags, money and phones.

My physical health is not stable either...I still have problems with my bladder. I still feel the urge to urinate every time! In hospital, it was worse off. I'd urinate on myself...urine would just drool on its own, but now I feel the urge to urinate, although the urge still comes too often!

Irregular menstrual periods are another set of challenges I now have to live with, especially agonizing period pains!

Although the bodily weaknesses and pains have troubled me a lot, but what pains me most about Ebola is the financial mess it has brought to my life.

I've spent a lot of money in the course of fighting Ebola. As I speak now, I am completely broken, financially.

I've had to take loans and sell some of my belongings, including a parcel of land to raise some funds to treat my recurrent health problems!!

5 DAUGHTER AS MOTHER'S HUSBAND

This is the story of a young business woman in her early twenties caught in the quagmire of Ebola. Her story reflects how an Ebola epidemic can distort people's realities in ways that are hard to comprehend!

A strange illness struck a week after we buried my little niece - my late brother's baby who'd died under mysterious circumstances! My little niece was found dead by her mother when she returned home from the garden a short distance away.

The little child was well and sound asleep before her mother, my sister-in-law, headed out to the garden at the edge of the forest nearby to keep away the predatory chimpanzees and monkeys from our food crops!

Still unsure of what had killed her; we buried my little niece the following day! A week later, her mother, my sister-in-law got sick. Her condition deteriorated rapidly and she also died a few days later! But before she died, she'd complained of very severe fever, headache. She also vomited a lot and reported passing lots of bloody diarrhea!

In line with our culture, we took my sister-in-law's

body for burial at her parents' home! A feud later erupted between the two families about her mysterious death. Her relatives wondered how their daughter could die within such a short time without us notifying them of her illness.

From their arguments, it was apparent that her family didn't believe us when we told them that she'd died of natural causes. They suspected that our family had played a role in causing her death. They were so upset that they warned us of dire consequences to come! From then onwards, we were sure that a "troubled future" lay ahead!

Less than a fortnight after the burial of my sister-law, I also became sick! I'd relentless headache, backache, fever and a strange sense of weakness. I decided to go to a nearby clinic. After treatment, the relief was temporary.

And the following week, nearly everyone in my household became ill - children and adults alike! "How could we all become ill at the same time?" we wondered! "Could this be the "catastrophe" our in-laws promised?" we asked ourselves!

This strange illness made our minds to go wild, as we imagined all sorts of possibilities! It was clear that the sick weren't responding to treatment anymore. And so we were convinced that the in-laws had executed their threat of a "*troubled future*". "The in-laws must've sent us evil spirits", we concluded! We were convinced because everyone had similar symptoms: grade fever; headache and vomiting!

With the two deaths and nearly every other person sick, we decided to take all the sick family members for special healing prayers at the shrine of a locally renowned *prophet*. This healer had earned himself a reputation for dealing with spiritual matters decisively, including witchcraft! We were thus convinced that the *prophet's* healing prayers would effectively counter the deaths caused by the spirits.

We then arranged to take all the sick for spiritual cleansing at the *prophets'* prayer palace, except one of my sisters who was five months pregnant. But shortly before we set off to the prayer palace, my sister began to bleed and so she was rushed off to nearby hospital because of bleeding. We thought the bleeding was due to an impending miscarriage!

Desperate to find an antidote for the *'evil spirits'*, we headed straight to the prayer palace in two car loads. When we arrived, we found hundreds of other people camped there as well, from both near and far off places! Surprisingly many had come from as far as Kenya, Congo and Rwanda. Like us, they'd come to seek spiritual healing for their problems as well!

Unfortunately the *prophet* wasn't available at the prayer palace. We had no option but to spend the night at his palace! As we waited, two of my brothers began to deteriorate rapidly. They started vomiting frank blood and passing bloody diarrhea! We became scared the more. We were worried we'd lose them - what a frightful day we had!

The following day we were scheduled to meet the *prophet*. But before the *prophet* could even lay his hands on my brothers to start praying for them, both of them died...right before his eyes! It must have been about 8:30am. These sudden and unusual deaths terrified everyone present!

Moved by how my brothers died – with blood oozing from their eyes and nose while vomiting profusely, the *prophet* told us that their disease did not seem "*spiritual*" in nature. He emphasized that the situation didn't call for his spiritual intervention; rather medical intervention would be the best!

Before long, the *prophet* instructed his driver to take all of us who were sick the hospital for formal medical care.

When we arrived, the doctors examined all of us and admitted those who were sick looking. And other family members proceeded to bury the two brothers who had died earlier in the morning. I was one of those admitted right away because I'd cough, fever and excruciating headache!

Just before we came to terms with the grief of losing two elder brothers on a single day, we were shocked with yet another bad news! A call came through from home that my expectant sister who was rushed to hospital the previous day bleeding had miscarried and later died due to bleeding.

What a terrible day…

I lost three family members in a single day!

The grief was unimaginable!

The visit to the *prophet's* palace was unsuccessful…

Neither was rushing my sister to the hospital proved useful! What a loss…the pain was almost unbearable!

When rumors of strange deaths in my family started doing the rounds, a team of health workers went home from the district hospital. It was decided that my entire family was to be hospitalized to facilitate close monitoring.

And so ambulances were sent home to bring the remaining family members for effective quarantine and observation in the isolation ward. When the remaining family members arrived, blood samples were taken from each one of them and swiftly sent to the national laboratory for analysis.

After about a week of waiting, the results came back! What came back was a shocker! "The disease you have been suffering from is Ebola" they told us! This news of Ebola outbreak shocked everyone including the health workers.

When I realized that the illness was caused by Ebola and not witchcraft as we'd earlier believed, I was terrified! What worried me most was the fact that whoever contracts Ebola usually has minimal chances of surviving the illness. And so I feared that my entire family would soon perish!

After a while, when the individual results were released, the outcome was both positive and negative for me and my family. The good news was that some relatives, although they looked sick, they were in fact already recovering from Ebola - they were already survivors. The bad news on the other hand was that a few others including myself tested positive for the deadly virus. This meant that there was a serious possibility of dying from Ebola in the near future!

For weeks, the remaining family members and I were quarantined in the isolation ward. We were given medications for symptoms of headache, body pains and diarrhea. And we waited to see what would happen to us! With time, some family members became better and were eventually discharged, while others deteriorated and died.

In total 9 family members perished…
It was such a great loss for us…unimaginable you'd say!

Luckily, despite the loss, I and a few family members survived - this was after an additional 3 weeks in the hospital. It is then that I was ready to be discharged home.

When I heard about going home, I couldn't hide my joy! It was an exciting day for me, a day I will live to remember! All seemed well as the surveillance team drove me home!

When I arrived home, I soon noticed that this feeling of elation would be short lived! I was rudely shocked when I noticed that my neighbors were unwilling to associate with us, notably my grand ma, my mum, my sister and a young niece! Only a few people weren't afraid of us…but most neighbors actively avoided us and refused to mix with us!

This open rejection by friends and distant family members was extremely depressing! "How can people be so unkind to us?" I would ask! I'd sometimes pray to God to touch their hearts so that they would stop avoiding us! I was desperate; I wanted to be accepted back into the fold!

All I wanted was to be treated like a normal human being with dignity and respect. It was heart wrecking that some people were deliberately treating us inhumanely. In spite of several assurances from health workers and political leaders that Ebola survivors weren't harmful, most people refused to abide by their counsel. Rather, they continued to ignore me and my family and openly rejected me and other family members at every opportunity that availed itself!

With no clear end of ostracism in sight, it became difficult to fend for my family. I couldn't work in my hair salon. I desperately needed to be accepted so that I could earn some money to buy provisions. I'd now become the head of the family. My elder brothers, sisters and my father had all perished in the previous months.

I desperately wanted people to feel free with me again. Our home which before long was always busy was deserted; even grass covered the path to our home, as stigma skyrocketed, as if we're dead!

When I realized that people were afraid of us, I told my household that we should confine ourselves to staying at home until the fear diminished significantly. Although alone and isolated, we decided to live a near-normal life as much as our circumstances allowed. We'd stay close to one another, consoling one another, for about three months.

Although rejected by neighbors and relatives, we decided to stand strong. As the oldest surviving daughter of the family, I had to constantly comfort the rest, especially my mother and others under my care.

Despite the challenges we faced, I couldn't allow anyone, especially my mother to become hopeless! I was particularly determined to take care of my mom just as my daddy willed before he died!

I remember to this day when he whispered, "My daughter I know I won't make it, and you now have to be your mothers' 'husband'". From that moment onwards, I knew I'd become an heir to my father! This meant that whatever my mother and others under my care needed, I'd to struggle to provide, like my dad would've if he were alive! Soon I realized this obligation wasn't easy at all!

While I tried to be brave and faced the numerous challenges head on, at times I'd get destructed and become engrossed in thoughts. I'd sometimes find myself weeping! I'd cry because of the so many difficulties and the loss of my close relatives. I'd sometimes imagine that if I hadn't lost my brothers and sisters I wouldn't be suffering as much! Whenever I felt overwhelmed I would stop and cry until I gathered enough strength to face life's puzzles again!

I remembered crying bitterly when the local FM radio station falsely and repeatedly announced about more deaths in my home. What exasperated me most is when they falsely announced that my mother and I had died! I couldn't understand why they wanted us dead after all we'd gone through as a family. I nearly suffered a nervous breakdown as the pressure mounted. It became increasingly intolerable. I couldn't bear these false announcements; I even developed high blood pressure!

The allegations of my death made me lose all my salon customers, because most people thought that I'd perished. They would describe me as the 'salon lady' who died; creating fear in my customers and eventually killing my business. The radio announcements were distressing…, one day I had to make an emergency call home to clarify if my mother had indeed died as was being aired at the time!

At another point, the local FM radio announced that my grandmother had hanged herself, when this wasn't the case! Such false announcements stressed me a great deal! These and related acts only made my situation worse and only heightened my anxiety. These announcement and declarations stretched me to breaking point. We were pushed to a stage where we couldn't take any more stress! And so to just keep sane, my mother and I decided to switch off the radios, preferring media blackout!

Days later, when we switched the radios back on, the discussions about my family continued. I could no longer bear these taunts and falsehoods. One morning I went straight to the radio station and questioned them as to why they don't verify their information before making public announcements! I left them with no doubt that we were upset by their behavior. I even gave them my cell phone numbers and urged them to please verify whatever information they have about my family before making unfair pronouncements about me or my family members!

From then on, they would first seek confirmation from us before they made any of such public pronouncements. Luckily they heeded! When my aunt died a few weeks later, due to causes, unrelated to Ebola, they first consulted me before making an announcement about her demise. Finally, a radio presenter had at least made us feel better!

Part of the attitude change as we noticed with the radio presenter came as a result of relentless efforts by health teams and local politicians. These officials tirelessly advised the masses that survivors and their close family members weren't dangerous and shouldn't be feared! Although these efforts started way before the epidemic was declared over, the campaigns began to bear fruit several months after the outbreak was officially declared ended!

After three months, some neighbors and distant relatives began to beat the odds. Slowly, they started visiting us. It seemed the fear in the community had gradually begun to diminish following several weeks of sensitization talks in villages and over local FM radios. These talks appeared to have gradually changed people's attitudes and behaviors!

Despite the relative change of people's attitudes towards us, the suffering my family and I endured is still fresh in my mind. It was so bad that I'm still terrified whenever I hear the mention of the word *Ebola*. The news of Ebola still fills me with awe and shock, often leaving me moribund!

Also despite months of health education, the community is still not very easy with me. I still don't have sufficient customers for my salon business. And so my zeal for the business has diminished a lot. What discourages me most is that I often spend days, without getting a single customer, and yet I still have to pay rent for the property!

However, despite several disappointments I decided that I'll not give up. And being the heir to the family, whenever I feel low and discouraged, I tell myself, "If I don't persist in the salon work, where will I find money to look after the people under my care?" Whenever I remind myself of such stark realities, I always find myself strong once again; ready to move on, never giving up in the face of adversity!

To further boost my mental energy, I would tell myself that I have to work extremely hard since, I am now my mother's husband, my younger sister's father and too my daughter's grandfather, let alone being caretaker of my grandmother and my niece who are orphaned by Ebola".

And these days when I reflect upon my experience with Ebola, it is clear that Ebola is one of the worst diseases, comparable to no other! And when I think about my family situation, I feel worried because we still have to endure physical difficulties as well as economic challenges.

These difficulties notwithstanding, I am still exceedingly grateful to God for healing me from Ebola. I also thank the health workers who treated in hospital. I am grateful as well to the health workers who came home regularly to counsel us...we greatly appreciated their effort.

What I remember most is how the various teams explained to us how to be careful with ourselves and others and this helped us a lot. Unlike many others, these health workers never feared us and for this I'm exceedingly happy! In fact their actions made us feel we were normal human beings. This support helped us to move along the unpleasant road of recovery, after losing so many relatives!

6 COPING THROUGH DESTRUCTION

This is the story of a Grandmother who lost nine members of her family within a month! Exceedingly distraught and desperate to erase the memories of the deceased, she embarks on an unusual remedy...to destroy the houses where the deceased relatives lived!

I began to feel unwell slightly over a week after my husband died of an unknown disease. For over two weeks, he'd had high fever, headaches, and aches and bled a lot before he died. No one knew what was causing the high fevers, diarrhea, body pain, vomiting and the bleeding!

Even though I was the one taking care of him, I wasn't sure what had killed my husband. I only came to know that he could've died of Ebola after more than two weeks. We buried him without knowing precisely what killed him.

Initially, when I fell sick, there was nothing unusual with how I felt. It was the usual fever and headache which I always had whenever I had malaria or something of sorts. And so I took fever tablets and anti-malarial meds from home. But after days of home based treatment it was clear the meds were not working as the symptoms continued.

As I struggled with fever, cough and headache, two of my sons and my daughter also became ill. For days, they complained of fever, headache and joint aches. Again just like me, they never responded to the medications. Just like me their symptoms worsened by the day. We're worried!

Perplexed and unsure of the illness we concluded the disease could have had a spiritual dimension. And so we began searching for options where we could get spiritual healing. After a while we settled for a renowned prophet known to heal all manner of illnesses of spiritual nature, like sorcery, through special prayers at his "sanctuary".

But before we could set off to the prayer place, my daughter who was pregnant began bleeding. She had been complaining of fever and headache throughout the past week. We had to immediately arrange transport to take her to a nearby hospital for emergency medical attention. As my daughter was being rushed to the hospital, I and five other family members started off to the prophet's "shrine".

After hours of travel along dusty roads, we arrived at the prayer palace. Regrettably we didn't find the prophet at home that evening. So we'd to spend the night there! In the late evening, my two sons began to complain of acute pain in the abdomen. Both started vomiting blood and passing bloody diarrhea. What a terrible sight it was! People at the prophet's place wondered in bewilderment. What a sight it was!

An emergency call was sent to the prophet about the dire state of my sons! Unfortunately he was stuck some kilometers away and wouldn't be back till later. And so an appointment was fixed for him to see my sons first thing the next morning. The following day, as my two sons were being lined up alongside other sick people for the prophet to him to lay hands, the unthinkable happened! I couldn't imagine: my two sons started convulsing and vomiting!

When the prophet saw this he immediately told me that my sons were not suffering from anything spiritual.

Rather, he argued their disease needed medical attention. He was quick to suggest that we should go to the hospital right away. He offered a minibus to facilitate our transit. Even before we could board the cars to travel to the district hospital, which was about two hours away, my two sons deteriorated further and died right there...before every one!

At the death of the two sons, the prophet offered another car - one to take other sick family members to the hospital and the other to carry the bodies of the two sons and a few other family members including myself back to our home. In the end, the sick family members were taken to hospital, while myself and a few others returned home for burial!

When we arrived home and the news spread that two of my sons had died. The villagers were frightened. The situation was even worsened when news came in later that afternoon that my elder daughter who was taken to hospital the previous day due to bleeding had also died! With three deaths in a single day - pandemonium erupted!

In great hurry, people started leaving our village; for fear that the strange disease that had by then killed six members of my family would also spread to them. And when I saw people running away and escaping to lands far off, I asked myself, "Where can I run to?" I felt sorry for them. But unlike them, I swore never to abandon the home were my husband and the children and grandchildren were buried!

The death of my husband, children and in-law, one after another, left the entire neighborhood in shock and awe! They asked questions like, "Why would so many people die like this in a single family?" My loss was mind boggling as people tried to understand the cause of the mysterious deaths – which were unprecedented and incomprehensible!

The rumors of strange deaths in my home spread rapidly. It was being discussed everywhere - along the village paths, and over counters in drinking places and on the local FM radio! The rumors were so widespread. A few days after my daughter and other family members were admitted to hospital, some health workers came home to investigate if the rumors of unexplained deaths in my home were true!

When the team arrived and saw the graves, they decided that everyone in the family whether sick or not who had been in contact with the other deceased relatives should be taken to the hospital for close monitoring. And later day, everyone in my home was taken to the district hospital. When we arrived, we joined some of the family members who had been admitted after being referred by the prophet.

The following day, we were told that samples of blood and stool would be taken from us and sent to the city for testing. Up to this time, they still hadn't discovered what the strange illness was and so the investigations continued. And so we waited to find out what was killing us - my husband, my children and other adults as well! We couldn't come with any real idea of the cause of the deaths!

Within a week the results were back! The findings were shocking! We'd been infected by the deadly Ebola virus! Luckily for me, the test results showed that I was no longer ill. In fact physically, I had already started eating and the symptoms of fever and general body pains had subsided.

What was rather strange is that when I was told that I'd survived Ebola; I wasn't sure whether to feel happy or sad, I was confused! While I knew Ebola usually kills its victims mercilessly, and somehow my survival meant I was among the lucky few, I wasn't excited much! Clearly, my happiness had been dampened by the deaths in my home!

Thinking about my situation months later, maybe I would have shouted out loud in joy, if there was reason for me to be happy then! The pain of losing nine close relatives - my grandchildren, children, daughters-in-law and my husband of 40 years were still fresh in my mind. With such loss so fresh, I would ask myself, "Is there any real reason for me to be happy?" "What's there to celebrate anyway?" I'd ask!

After undergoing counseling in hospital for a few more days I was eventually released to go back home, while the rest of the family members who were sick were detained. When I arrived home from hospital, everything about me and my life changed overnight and drastically!

Neighbors and close relatives began to shun my home. This avoidance continued close to a year despite radio announcements and assurances from health workers and our local politicians.

Ever since the deaths occurred and people ran away from our village, most people would openly ostracize us; me and a few of the surviving members of the family. In fact I dare say that the last time people came to my home freely, was when they came for the funeral of the first few relatives - my granddaughter, her mother and my husband.

Once the deaths increased and Ebola was confirmed, people started shunning my family. The deaths of my two sons and my daughter on a single day exacerbated the already tense situation! From this moment on, the ostracism intensified!

Ever since that time, unlike in the past, neighbors and relatives became reluctant to come home. They'd simply pass by and avoided to set a foot on my compound. Of my close relations, only my uncle would come home to bring us supplies, since we couldn't get anything from neighbors!

The shunning made me feel very lonely, since most of the older children and my husband had perished and no grownups were visiting us. With time, these difficulties notwithstanding, I decided that I wouldn't allow the deaths and the community's negative behavior to ruin me. "I've to be strong despite these difficulties", I'd often insist. The few remaining children, especially the heir to my late husband always comforted and counseled me. Although young, she always acted like an elderly person. She was instrumental in helping me return to a fairly "normal" life!

And so months after the deaths and in spite of the social isolation, I continued to live a 'near normal' life as much as possible. "I can't continue to live in misery", I reasoned! I also told myself that I'd move forward despite the loss of my loved ones and the shunning. I told myself that I would construct my life back and start from a new!

Strangely after some time, some of the few relatives and friends who managed to come home advised me to abandon my present home. They encouraged me to move to another location so that I'd forget my troubles! They reasoned that if I continued to live in my present home I would feel sad every day and would become depressed!

But I refused! I would tell them that whilst it's true the home reminded me of the many deaths, I promised my heir-daughter that I would never abandon and flee from this home..., the home of my 40 years marriage, where I've buried my children, their wives and my own husband! "These people buried here are my loved ones, how could I possibly I leave their memories behind?" I would reiterate!

As time went by, my resolve to be strong slowly began to dissipate. Although I vowed to be strong against the challenges, the shunning and stigma were steadily wearing me down. I was particularly disturbed when people I considered friends or allies engaged in ostracizing us. Even the rumors and memories of the loved ones all began to break me down emotionally. Of these, what troubled me most were the empty houses left by the deceased relatives!

Whenever I set my eyes on the houses where children once lived, I would feel a violent churn inside me and the image of the deceased would instantly flash through my mind. These empty houses always brought me bitter memories. The flashing images of the deceased were catastrophic! "God why did this happen to me?" I would lament wearily. My compound was always full and now no more, because everyone is gone! The sense of aloneness persisted!

I always felt tormented whenever I saw the empty houses. The unusual eerie feeling around my compound kept coming back, whenever I glanced at the empty houses! I would be reminded of how warm my household was and the old memories kept flashing through my mind. I would ask "Why did this happen to me?" Life became intolerable!

And when I could no longer bear the haunting feeling of loss, the creepy feeling and the constant heartache, I decided to destroy all the houses where my children and their spouses once lived. I destroyed all buildings that reminded me of my loss. These empty houses had become an awful symbol of my loss and this hurt me so bad. I thought I'd be less haunted if I demolished the houses!

A few months later, I discovered I was wrong...the lasting relief I sought didn't come fully. It was short lived - once in a while the perturbing images of the deceased would flash through my mind, although less often, but they're present!

To this day, when I reflect about this whole experience, I still feel a lot of pain in my heart. But with nothing much to do about it, I regain my strength and try to forget about it. I sometimes feel angry, because the way we used to live before Ebola was not how it is today. I still feel very lonely!

These days, there are barely any people in my compound — quite the opposite of the home that was always full of people- cheerfully noisy! Mine was a home where people grew together in joy and harmony; a home that made me a proud wife, mother and grandmother.

We lived a very contented and happy and lively life together. But today, the compound is empty and the home is quiet and ghostly!

❧❧

7 SURVIVING EBOLA - VICTORS, VICTIMS AND THE SCARS

Life after Ebola is like a double edged sword - with both negative and positive effects. For some, life becomes progressively better as they attain a higher meaning of life; while others face a plethora of negative experiences!

What happens next after an Ebola patient leaves the isolation unit matters a lot. It is what they hear, see or sense that drives them to conclude and consider whether their experience is positive or negative overall! What happens within survivors' bodies and around them especially how they're received is a critical determinant!

From Light to Transient Shadows

When survivors are discharged from hospital the initial feeling is that of euphoria and jubilation. For some, this joyous period lasts for a long time, while for others it quickly turns ugly. This is especially so when they encounter the seemingly endless list of challenges. For most survivors these challenges are both internal and external to them! These relate to physical, social, psychological, economic as well as spiritual difficulties!

The physical difficulties survivors have to endure include episodes of excruciating bone and muscle pains that come and go...for some in a cyclical manner. These symptoms severely weaken survivors and make their lives miserable! Whenever such difficulties appear, survivors' life styles get altered - they are often forced to cope with new limitations!

The social difficulties start as survivors are publicly rejected, ostracized and stigmatized needlessly, leaving them emotionally sore! This rejection starts early during outbreaks, often beginning with news of an outbreak, and continues several months after the outbreak ends! It seems the *"pain"* of rejection is more pronounced if survivors are abandoned by individuals they consider friends or family.

The psychological struggles on the other hand relate to the constant worry, the unending stress and ironically, the lingering possibility of death from the aftereffects of Ebola. Survivors also experience mental stress from the rampant social isolation and open rejection which lingers unceasingly! With time, the seemingly unending physical, social as well as the economic challenges weigh heavy on survivors' shoulders; leaving them exhausted emotionally!

The economic difficulties experienced may be attributed to different reasons. First, survivors often have financial difficulties, in part due to their diminished ability to function socially and physically. Socially, the widespread stigma means some survivors are unable to return to their jobs. And physically, the after effects of Ebola such as the chronic pain or poor hearing and eye sight leave survivors debilitated!

These limitations significantly lessen their ability to find and maintain work, because as with most economic endeavors, good health is a must. In essence, this poor health prevents them from operating at their best!

Another often unintended economic difficulty results from the sudden loss of property as a consequence of the *"destroy the source"* infection prevention policy usually implemented by the surveillance teams. This protocol involves burning, burying or spraying of suspects' personal effects like beddings, furniture and clothes. It is the resulting loss of property that contributes to survivors' financial misery.

While affected families are somewhat compensated by health authorities and the central government, frequently the funds allotted for such compensation does not fully cover the costs of the personal property that was destroyed.

The final and yet critical challenge survivors have to navigate through is finding the meaning in their suffering. This constitutes a major element of spiritual difficulty. These seemingly endless problems forces survivors to ask themselves repeatedly questions such as, "*Why me*?" "Why did I survive?" and "Why did my children die?" and so on!

Such meaning making struggles often linger on in the minds of survivors for months and even years. These mental processes may be interpreted as survivors' ways of coming to terms with their pains including social isolation!

From Darkness to Light - Living as Victors!

When survivors emerge victorious, it probably means they have surmounted the plethora of physical, social, economic and spiritual challenges related to their association with Ebola. It means they have moved from '*living in darkness* to *living in light*'! Despite the numerous challenges they often have to deal with, "victors" are habitually grateful for their survival and are amazingly good at *"picking up their pieces"* and then moving right back!

Some survivors are extraordinary; they find life after Ebola more meaningful compared to their past life. Such survivors transcend the negative experiences encountered and transform them to find more meaning in their suffering in very strange ways! In effect such survivors become "super victors", for being able to flourish after catastrophe!

From Dusk to Darkness - Living as Victims!

When survivors fail to overcome the numerous challenges associated with Ebola infection, many end up feeling and behaving as "victims". Characterized by acceptance of defeat and continuous episodes of sadness and self-pity, such survivors sometimes end up with chronic depression. Quite often, "victims" are survivors who receive little support or those who are abandoned by their relatives!

While such survivors ably overcame Ebola at physiological level, regrettably they fail to overcome the difficulties after hospitalization. Instead they withdraw from others and remain isolated for months! A few others become "super victims": they voluntarily choose to die after initially struggling to survive! What a contradiction you may say!

8 EPILOGUE
WHERE IT ALL ORIGINATED

In the each of the five personal stories, you hear a constant echo of *"I don't know I had Ebola!"* These statements clearly show how individuals and their families struggled to place Ebola in contexts that may've allowed them to trace the origins of the disease. As shown in figure 1, these two outbreaks (Gulu 2000, Kibale 2012) occurred in a geographical region that has for the last 40 years shown its proneness to Ebola outbreaks. In fact both outbreaks occurred in an area that is close to where the world's first recorded epidemic of Ebola occurred in 1976, following concurrent outbreaks in Nzara in the Sudan and Yambuku in Eastern Democratic Republic of the Congo, then Zaire!

These areas are linked by continuous vegetation cover and are part of the equatorial belt consisting of tropical rain forests, thick bush belts and grasslands where a variety of mammals co-exist especially our *"cousins"*, the gorillas, chimpanzees and monkeys. This geographical reality appears to aid the sporadic outbreaks of Ebola in this wider region thanks to the close interaction between the local populations and the non-human primates, especially these *"cousins"* who are hunted for food and medicinal portions!

On their own too, these *cousins* of ours frequently come to human settlements to *"revenge"* on crops like corn, peanuts, cassava and potatoes, especially those cultivated at the edge of forests and thickets. In addition to the chimpanzees and the like, locals living near the forests also get exposed to a variety of bats, the *undisputed* natural reservoirs of a number of viral diseases like Ebola, Rabies and Marburg.

Indeed scientific studies conducted in Uganda, Gabon and the Democratic Republic of the Congo have firmly linked filovirus, one of which is the notorious Ebola virus to some varieties of the African fruit bats. In sub Saharan Africa, these bruit bats have been able to transmit filoviruses to humans as a result of frequent interaction with the locals.

In the recent past, outside Africa, the role of these bats in human disease transmission came to light in 2008, after a 40-year-old Dutch tourist, according to the World health organization, became infected and later died of Marburg infection, after returning from Uganda in June 2008. As part of her excursion, she had made two trips to "python caves" in Maramagambo Forest, an extensive rain forest which is part of Queen Elizabeth National Park (QENP) in the far West of Uganda, bordering Kibale district, where the 2012 Ebola outbreak occurred and where the stories of four of the five survivors continues to unfold!

In this region several studies have implicated fruits bats in the transmission of Marburg viruses, the closest associate of Ebola virus. These conclusions are based on ecological studies that consistently show that about 5% of the fruit bats in Kitaka mines in the nearby Kamwenge district (see map) had evidenced of prior Marburg virus infestation. It has thus been confirmed that some bat species in western Uganda are reservoirs for filoviruses!

Like in the case of the Dutch tourist, exposure to these deadly agents of filoviruses occurs both directly and indirectly. First, these bats often feed on the same fruits as the locals….among them bananas, mangoes and guavas which grow in abundance in and around the forests and the thickets. Second, these bats are also eaten by the locals as delicacies. Therefore, if a particular bat has the virus, an innocent roast of a bat for an early dinner may precipitate a full scale epidemic. A third way, little of which is often said in literature is the fact that when the usually rich "bellies" of the forest fruits dry up, especially during the drier seasons of the year, these bats are drawn to people's houses for food, creating another window for direct contact with humans, thus increasing the possibility of viral infections!

As I interacted with these communities, they were reports of bats hanging around the villages in large numbers especially in the evenings during dry seasons. There were also reports of incidences where a few people had been attacked by bats and sliced with razor sharp teeth, leaving small, gaping wounds. These tales are familiar to stories of villagers in the Amazonian villages in Brazil and Peru, Latin America, where attacks by a particular type of bats, commonly referred to as the "blood-drinking vampire" bats has led to rabies outbreaks, another serious viral infection.

The stories of the villagers in Kibale district, especially where the 2012 outbreak occurred resonate well with real life stories of vampire bat attacks typically occurring when the victim is asleep. The bats use heat sensors to find a victim's veins and make a small tear in the skin using their razor sharp teeth. The bats then sit down quietly for *dinner;* and lap up the oozing blood as the ultimate payment for their ingenious efforts, transmitting diseases in the process!

The blood sucking bats have a potent anticoagulant in their saliva, referred to as *"Draculin"* that thins the victim's blood and keeps the blood from clotting, so it keeps flowing until the blood tap runs dry! In addition to the anticoagulant, another chemical in their saliva numbs the victim's skin so it doesn't wake up, and this allows each bat to gorge up on the evening meal...pretty undisturbed, drinking about a tablespoon of blood within half an hour.

Such human-bat interactions although rare, do occur. The 2012 Ebola outbreak in Kibale in Western Uganda seems to have begun after such contact with bats, through inferences drawn from the description of the villagers' in the index family. While conducting one to one interviews in home where this epidemic began, I was told by the survivors that the baby, whose death heralded what eventually, became an Ebola outbreak had her skin sliced and the blood *"sucked out"* by unknown crawling animals!

The family suspected the baby's hand could have been bitten and her blood sucked by a small blood sucking mammal, probably a bat, capable of crawling through the ventilators. This was because the door remained properly shut even when the baby's mother returned. The baby had been put to sleep before her mother headed off to her garden a short distance away, at the edge of the forest, to keep monkeys and chimpanzees at bay!

Upon returning home, she reportedly found the baby dead...and astonishingly pale, with a clean cut wound on the back of her left hand...and nothing more. The baby remained well covered exactly how her mother had left her: what was new was the wound. After returning from the garden the baby's mother was prompted to check on the baby by her mother in-law, the baby's grandmother!

Apparently the grandmother was concerned why the baby hadn't woken up. Besides, the baby appeared to have slept far longer than she usually did! The discovery by the mother about the baby's death astonished everyone at home. Stunned by her death, the baby's mother and later other family members examined the baby's cut wound over and over again...before burying her the following day!

And when I pressed about animals they knew could have made such cuts, the villagers told me they had heard that when a rare type of bats was very hungry, they would attack and feed on human and animal blood. When I heard this, I quickly connected the missing link! I then asked myself…"Could it be that the baby was attacked by a bunch of hungry bats while she slept?, And, "Can a bunch of hungry bats suck out so much blood and leave a baby pale"? Grippingly, the answer to both questions was "yes!"

This revelation inspired me to extensively review literature about bats and to my surprise; I found that it was actually possible that the baby might have been "sucked dry" by a "gang" of hungry bats. These small mammals could have sneaked through the ventilators, located the baby's veins in the exposed hand, sliced her skin and lapped up her blood!

Why did I believe this? Just like Daniel Riskin of Cornell University, USA is quoted as saying…"bats can suck up to 10 millimeters (0.34 oz.) of blood at a single sitting within a period of 30 minutes". This is a very significant amount of blood for a 3 month old infant whose total blood volume is about 400ml. A hearty "suck up" by hungry bats means considerable amount of blood could have been consumed!

Knowing that such bats feed in groups, the sheer volume of blood lapped up would mean that the bats were capable of leaving the baby instantly anemic. This possibility is further supported by the possibility of continuous bleeding as a result of anticoagulant activity promoted by the bats' saliva. It is possible that the anticoagulation activity of the saliva may have persisted even after the bats sneaked away!

From a physiological view point, it can be concluded that most probably, the loss of blood resulting from the direct (lapping) and indirect action (post feeding bleeding) of the bats meant the blood lost may have exceeded the lethal 40% mark. This sudden loss of blood may've precipitated *'hypovolemic shock'*, a medical emergency characterized, internally, by decreased blood pressure, high pulse, and externally, sweaty, cool and pale appearance.

Thinking about the little baby, the sudden loss of blood is most probably what impeded her fragile heart from pumping sufficient blood to her body, eventually leading to her death. These recollections made me to conclude that the most probable reason for the baby's death and the usual paleness was the end result of a massive "suck up", by a gang of hungry bats that occurred as she slept that evening!

Another interesting turn of events I noted from their stories is that the baby's mother died two weeks after this episode. Before her death, she reportedly complained of Ebola like symptoms, namely headache, fever, vomiting and then blood oozing from her gums and mouth just before she died. This made me to conclude that this "little monsters", the bats, did not only "suck up" the baby's blood, but also contaminated the baby's cut wound with the Ebola virus!

I concluded that the transmission of the viruses from the little baby to her mother and others most probably occurred as her mother and others examined the "neatly cut flap of skin" on the back of her left hand. Also the handling of the corpse according to traditional burial rites may have provided another opportunity for the transmission of the viruses from the "*flap*" to others.

This repeated direct contact with the baby's cut skin would eventually prove fatal...it almost led to the extermination of this index family! This mysterious illness that resulted from this incident led to the loss of 9 lives from one family, within a few weeks! Surprisingly, this incidence led to the mysterious death – which was later declared as an Ebola outbreak by the Ministry of Health!

PICTORIAL REMINISCENCE

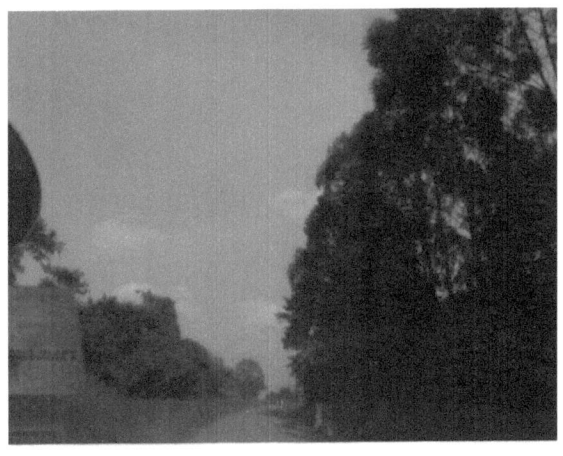

On the road- traveling to the index family home in Kibale district

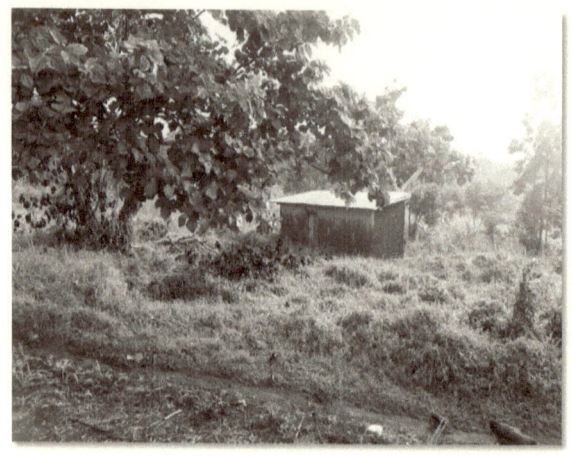

Abandoned - the house where the dead baby was discovered

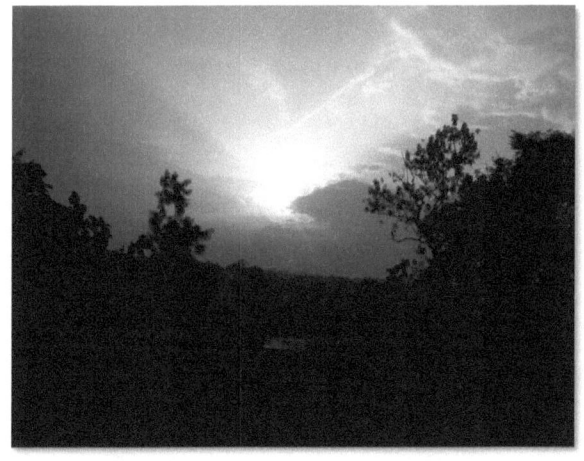

Spectacular- sunset from the home of the index family in Kibale district

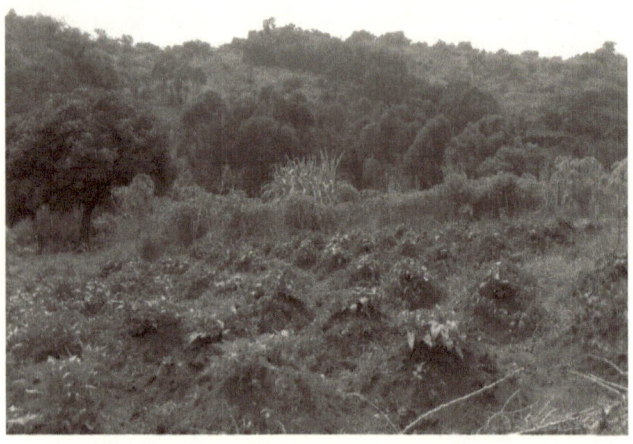

Mangos, potatoes, cassava and trees - ideal for human-animal interaction

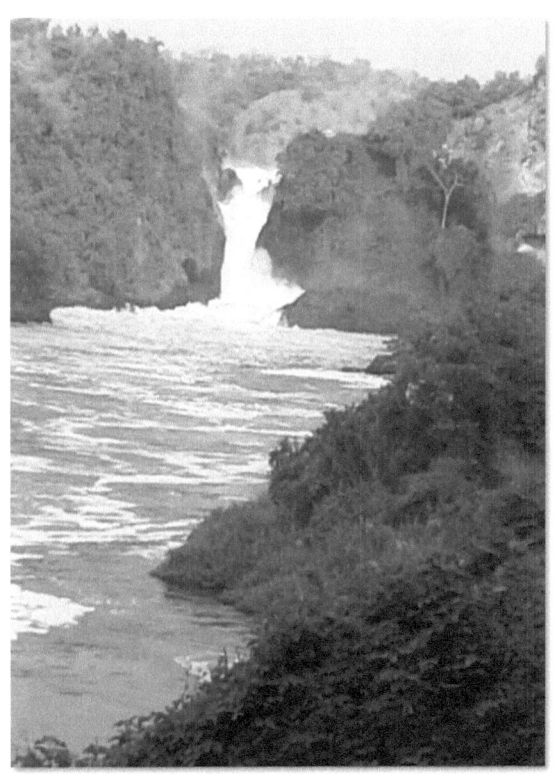

Scenic stopover - Murchison falls en route to Gulu for the interviews

GLOSSARY

Celsius- A unit of measurement for temperature, also known as centigrade, named after Swedish astronomer Anders Celsius, denoted as degrees Celsius (°C).

Clorox/Jik as known in Uganda is a chlorine based-sodium hypochlorite solution used for disinfecting and sterilizing; it kills bacteria, viruses and algae.

Coma - Is a state of unconsciousness that lasts for more than six hours, within which a person cannot be awakened, fails to respond to stimuli and can't speak, hear or move.

Disease-A condition when normal functioning of the body is hindered or damaged and can lead to death.

Draculin-A glycoprotein found naturally in the saliva of "vampire" bats. It has very strong anticoagulation properties, with capacity to prevent blood clotting.

Ebola Hemorrhagic Fever- A severe disease that results from infection with a lipid-enveloped single stranded RNA virus causing shock and bleeding problems.

Ebola Virus- A single stranded RNA virus that causes shock and bleeding abnormalities in humans and primates leading to death in up to 90% of the cases.

Epidemic-Occurrence of a disease in a community in excess of normal expectations.

Fahrenheit-A unit of measurement for temperature developed by German physicist Daniel Fahrenheit, denoted by the symbol degrees Fahrenheit (°F)

Gulu district - A district in northern Uganda, famously known for the fighting between Ugandan army and his Lord's Resistance Army. It is also where Uganda's first Ebola outbreak occurred in 2000.

Hypovolemic shock -When there is decreased blood volume; frequently from blood loss due to bleeding, leading to very low blood volume, resulting in death.

Infection- Entry and development of an infectious agent in the body, leading to disease and possible death.

Intravenous therapy- IV in short, referred to as a drip, means infusing liquid substances directly into a person's vein using specially designed system of tubes and needles.

Isolation ward - A special ward within hospitals used to isolate and reduce the spread of infection in patients with infectious diseases such as tuberculosis.

Kampala- The capital and largest city in Uganda, located in the south of the country. It is Uganda most cosmopolitan city with an international population, popularly described as the "City of 7 Hills".

Kibale district- A district in Western Uganda named after its main town. It houses the world famous Kibale National Park, home of the *Red Colobus* monkey. The district has the highest diversity and concentration of primates in African continent and is magnate for primate research.

Lord's Resistance Army - Also known as the Lord's Resistance Movement. It is a militant "Christianist", movement, comparable to the "Islamist" extremist groups like the Boko Haram of Nigeria. It operated in northern Uganda and South Sudan and the Democratic Republic of the Congo, since 2005, with the aim of ruling Uganda according to the Judeo-Christian Ten Commandments.

Malaria- Is a mosquito-borne infectious disease caused by parasitic protozoans called Plasmodia. The symptoms include fever, fatigue, vomiting and headache.

Marburg virus- Is a virus belonging to the Filoviridae family like Ebola virus. It causes Marburg virus disease, a viral hemorrhagic fever in humans and nonhuman primates. The disease was first identified in the 1960s, following small outbreaks in Marburg and Frankfurt in Germany and Belgrade in Serbia.

Oral rehydration solution- abbreviated as ORS, is the solution that results from mixing water with sugar and salt for use in oral rehydration therapy.

Oral rehydration therapy - Abbreviated as ORT, it's a type of body fluid replacement frequently used for the treatment of dehydration. It entails drinking large volumes of water mixed with sugar and salt, while continuing to eat.

Outbreak-A sudden onset of a disease, usually greater than expected at a particular time and place. It may affect a small and localized group or thousands of people.

Rabies- Is a viral disease that causes severe inflammation of the brain in humans and other warm blooded animals, with symptoms of fever and tingling at the site of exposure followed by violent movements, uncontrolled excitement, fear of water, confusion, and loss of consciousness and eventually death. It is transmitted to human when an infected animal scratches or bites another animal or human.

Reservoir-Any person, animal, arthropod, plant, soil or substance, in which an infective agent normally lives and multiplies, using the host for their survival.

Surveillance of disease-The on-going systematic collection and analysis of data and provision of information which leads to action being taken to prevent and control spread of an infectious disease.

Surveillance team- A team that systematically collects and analyses data including tracking and reporting about individuals suspected to have an infectious disease.

Virus- Is a very tiny infectious agent that is only able to live inside a cell composed of the outer protective shell and inner part made of the genetic material.

ACKNOWLEDGMENTS

This book is a byproduct of years of formal research as part of my master's and doctoral research. It spans a period of over ten years of research and community service in two Ebola affected communities in Uganda, East Africa that experienced debilitating Ebola outbreaks in 2000 and 2012.

Although this book was never an objective of my formal academic endeavors, inevitably my interactions with the affected individuals planted in me the seeds of this book. And this would not have been possible without the encouragement and trust of Professors Rozzano Locsin and Dirk Van der Wal, my master's and doctoral advisors.

In a very special way I thank the survivors, young and old, men and women and their families in both Gulu and Kibale districts for allowing me into their lives. I am more than certain that without their acceptance to open their often *silenced* worlds to me; these *untold stories* would still have remained in the depths of their hearts. As I promised to each of them, I will endeavor to tell each of these stories with the deepest respect, in a manner that the world may come to know what it means to survive Ebola, a disease whose name continues to generate *goose* pimples and send cold chills down the spines of the bravest of *medics*.

In a particular way, I also thank Dr. Bongomin Bodo and Mr. Kefa Madira, each for selflessly leading me to the villages in Gulu and Kibale districts respectively in 2001 and 2013. It is their physical tutelage that gave me the opportunity to learn from and engage with *victims* of Ebola.

I wish to salute my parents for planting in me the seeds of resilience and hard work; and my siblings for their physical and moral support. In a very special way I thank my wife and children for the sacrifice and encouragement, without which this book, the first of a series seven would be in vain. And for this I thank you for bearing with me, "for loving my computer a lot"…just know that every day of my life, *I live for you!*

ABOUT THE AUTHOR

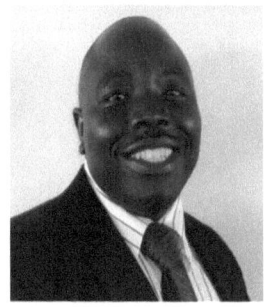

Gerald Amandu Matua, RN; PhD has over 15 years of experience in health care service, research, education and management. He has successfully leveraged this vast experience to become an author, speaker, career coach, and consultant in nursing and health professionals' education.

He regularly reviews journal articles and has authored highly cited articles, book chapters, technical reports and most recently the book *"Ebola: The Untold Stories of Survivors"*, which is part of book series that promote better understanding of the human side of Ebola outbreaks.

Dr. Amandu enjoys a remarkable career in nursing and health professional's education. He continues to participate in the training of nurses and midwives, physician assistants and doctors in universities in East Africa and the Middle East. Currently, Dr. Amandu lectures at Sultan Qaboos University in Oman, after serving as Senior Lecturer and Head of School of Nursing at International Health Sciences University, Uganda.

Dr. Amandu holds Bachelors and Masters Degrees in Nursing with a major in Education and Administration and a Doctorate in Health Studies. His research focuses on innovations in nursing and healthcare professionals' education, institutional leadership and management and infectious disease care, with special attention on the care of individuals and families affected by Ebola epidemics.

Dr. Amandu shares his life with wife Doreen and children Rozzano and Noela. In light moments he loves humor, music and likes to travel to new areas of the world.

www.ingramcontent.com/pod-product-compliance
Lightning Source LLC
Chambersburg PA
CBHW050429290526
45786CB00003B/1459